Allergy and Asthma Control—Naturally

Don't Just Cover up Symptoms with Drugs–
Attack the Root Causes with Safe,
Natural Alternatives!

Kent P. Kendall, M.B.A.

ISBN 0-7414-2838-5

Published by:

INFINITY PUBLISHING.COM

1094 New DeHaven Street, Suite 100
West Conshohocken, PA 19428-2713
Info@buybooksontheweb.com
www.buybooksontheweb.com
Toll-free (877) BUY BOOK
Local Phone (610) 941-9999
Fax (610) 941-9959

Printed in the United States of America

Printed on Recycled Paper

Published February 2006

DEDICATION

I wish to dedicate this book to my loving daughter, Heather, who will always be my little girl.

DISCLAIMER

Before we start our journey into the natural world of healing, here is the ubiquitous disclaimer:

This book is written for informational purposes only. The material in this book has not been evaluated by the Food and Drug Administration and is not intended to replace consultation with an appropriate health care provider. A qualified physician must do the diagnosis of a medical condition and recommend the appropriate initial treatment before alternative treatments can be considered. Do not discontinue taking your prescribed medications without your doctor's consent. The author, publisher and all reference sources shall have no liability to any person, persons, or legal entities that use any information contained in this book.

Don't let this legal talk scare you. Natural supplements are far safer than prescription drugs when used correctly. You will see the prescription drug statistics in Chapter 1.

TABLE OF CONTENTS

PREFACE

You may be wondering why did a guy with an engineering and information technology background write a medical-type book? When a family member was diagnosed with severe allergies and later with severe asthma, I found out that the medical profession could only offer prescription drugs to help ease the symptoms. One such drug retards growth in children. Other side effects include glaucoma and diabetes in some susceptible individuals.

For these reasons, I began to search for alternatives. The asthma drugs were almost as bad as the disease. I had already been studying alternative medicine since 1993, when I came across the use of Coenzyme Q10 for heart problems. It dramatically helped another member of my family. Since then, I have studied alternative medicine for many other conditions.

This book is the results of my quest to find natural supplements that will help control, and possibly eliminate, allergies and asthma. It's true that I am not a doctor, but I can report to you what researchers from around the world have found.

I wrote this book to be "middle of the road" in difficulty. Just listing supplements would make this work not much more than a laundry list like a lot of other alternative medicine books. You would not know if the supplements really worked or not. Instead, I have included scientific research studies that support my findings. The medical references will also give you credibility and leverage with your doctor when you discuss your situation. Some medical terminology is used, but you do not have to be a doctor to understand the material.

Recommended doses are listed after the symbol ◙. Cautions are flagged by the symbol ▼. The symbols make it easier to find this important information on a page. Appendix B gives helpful suggestions on when to take the various supplements. Many supplements depend on one or more additional supplements for absorption or effectiveness. Some supplements should not be taken at the same time because they interfere with each other. Appendix C allows you to record your own supplement plan. You can track your own progress by using the forms in Appendix D.

My family and I use many of the natural supplements discussed in this book. They have definitely helped us. I hope that you find this book informative and very useful in your "natural" fight against allergies and asthma.

Kent P. Kendal

CHAPTER 1

WHY GO NATURAL?

Why discuss natural treatments for asthma and allergies, anyway? Why not just use prescription or over-the-counter (OTC) drugs? Here are a few reasons:

- ✓ Prescription drugs are expensive
- ✓ Drugs usually have more adverse side effects
- ✓ Drugs only relieve symptoms – not underlying causes
- ✓ Natural treatments can sometimes effect a cure
- ✓ Natural treatments are usually much safer

Prescription drugs are not only expensive, but also have considerable adverse side effects. Corticosteroid drugs, for example, deplete the body of calcium, magnesium, potassium, and zinc. They may also increase the risk for cataracts.[1]

Even OTC antihistamine drugs cannot be used if you have certain conditions such as glaucoma, prostate problems, emphysema, or chronic bronchitis. Frequent acetaminophen users (6 –29 times per month) are more likely to have lung disease than non-users according to an English study. A study of more than 13,000 Americans also showed a 40% greater risk for asthma.[2] Acetaminophen is found in many medicines, including Tylenol®.

Prescription drugs have their place in getting critical symptoms under control rather quickly. They should be used with extreme caution, however. A study published in 1998 by the *Journal of the American Medical Association*, estimated that 106,000 hospital patients die each year from adverse drug reactions. Each year another 2,216,000 patients suffer permanent disability or require hospitalization from reactions to prescription drugs.[3] Remember, all these drugs have been approved by the *Food and Drug Administration* (FDA).

In August of 2005, a Texas jury found Merck & Co. liable for the death of a man who took the pain killer Vioxx. The jury awarded his widow $253 million. According to an article in the *Chicago Sun Times (August 21, 2005)*, one juror summed up the verdict by saying, "They needed to be held accountable for putting a drug out there that shouldn't be out there." Another juror said, "I want them to listen."

How many deaths and hospitalizations are reported each year from taking vitamins, minerals or other natural supplements correctly? It's near zero and yet the natural supplement industry is under continuous attack by the FDA, pharmaceutical companies (via unscientific studies) and certain members of congress. Why? You can't patent natural substances and make big bucks. Natural supplements are a threat to profits.

MY POSITION

I am all for the use of pharmaceuticals in emergency situations and when there are no alternatives available. They definitely have their place in medicine. I am against their use when safe, natural alternatives exist. This is especially true in the long-term management of an illness where adverse side effects can build up to intolerable levels and cause severe problems.

The FDA and the pharmaceutical companies should let the public have natural alternatives without harassment or legal roadblocks. They should put the health of people ahead of financial gains and power trips. The stakes are too high to do otherwise. We are talking about life and death!

THE NATURAL APPROACH

Natural nutrients have been used since ancient times to treat illnesses and conditions of all kinds. Modern society is gradually gravitating back toward natural or "alternative medicine" after seeing the general failings of conventional medicine. People want more than to have symptoms reduced at the expense of suffering side effects that are as bad as, or worse, than their ailment. Rarely are they actually healed; consequently, they seek help in less traditional medicine.

Natural supplements may take considerably longer to work and are not suitable for emergency situations. They are, however, more desirable for the long-term management of asthma and allergies. Drug alternatives are usually much safer because they occur in nature and can react in our bodies in a more natural way as compared to man-made, or synthetic drugs.

Both pharmaceuticals and natural supplements have a place in the treatment of asthma and allergies, but this book will focus on the natural supplements. Most of these natural alternatives have research studies to support their use.

Many different natural supplements are covered in this book. Why not just present one alternative? The answer is that each person is different and will respond differently to various treatments. What works dramatically for one person may be a dismal failure for another person. You have to experiment to find what works for you.

No substance will work 100% of the time on 100% of the people. Neither will pharmaceuticals. If a substance is effective 25% of the time, is it not worth a try? Combining natural supplements often increases your chances of being helped. Sometimes supplements have a synergistic effect. One supplement may be a co-factor for another. One may depend on another for absorption, activation or increased effect. These things will be covered later in more detail.

Don't give up! Keep trying and give the supplements enough time. Natural supplements often require considerable time to take full effect. The shortest time have I ever experienced was eight days. Most substances will take weeks or months. Some take a year. The Coenzyme Q10 cited in the preface took 12 weeks, but it was definitely worth it.

Patients with severe cases of allergy or asthma may never be able to completely eliminate dependence on pharmaceuticals, but they may be able to reduce the dosages. Even that would be worthwhile.

You may be wondering why I grouped asthma and allergies together. The two are highly related. Allergy is an inflammatory condition and asthma is a chronic inflammation of the airways. Persons with severe allergies are at risk for developing allergy-induced asthma. A second type of asthma is exercise-induced asthma. Both types are covered in this book. Fortunately, many of the natural supplements discussed alleviate both allergies and asthma.

One other thing worth mentioning is that using the supplements listed in this book may give you more than allergy or asthma relief. Other serious conditions, such as heart disease, arthritis and cancer, may be helped. Many diseases have an inflammation connection. Therefore, you are actually getting a lot more for your money with more safety. Can pharmaceuticals make that claim?

RESEARCH STUDY CAVEATS

Many of the natural approaches that follow have research studies listed as references. Just a word of caution about meta-analysis, which is an attempt to arrive at a conclusion by applying statistical analysis to scientific studies by grouping them in various ways. How you arbitrarily group data and how you use statistics determines the outcome. Meta-analysis is NOT an original, controlled scientific study.

Recently, a study contradicted the positive benefits of vitamin E that other studies have shown. The study is seriously flawed. The "researchers" concluded that those taking over 400 IU per day of vitamin E had a 0.48% increase in death rate. Sounds bad, right? Wrong! The authors arbitrarily assigned a very small group of people, who were already chronically ill, to the high dose group. They admitted that they did not know how healthy individuals would be affected.[4] For a detailed analysis of the study and all of its flaws, visit the following web site: http://www.vrp.com/art/1647.asp.

They also never addressed the quality of life the higher dose subjects might have had because of vitamin E. They only tracked mortality. They never documented the types of vitamin E that were consumed. Was it synthetic, natural alpha-tocopherol, or mixed, natural tocopherols? Was it taken with other vitamins and minerals?

It's like studying people who died of lung cancer who used cigarette lighters. You find a high statistical association between use of cigarette lighters and lung cancer. Can you conclude that carrying a pocket lighter causes lung cancer? Of course, not! Association does not mean causation!

Many people that die of lung cancer are smokers. Many used cigarette lighters to light up. They could have used matches, instead. The cigarettes caused the lung cancer – not the cigarette lighters; therefore, you cannot conclude that the use of cigarette lighters causes lung cancer.

So, just be careful when sensational articles appear that refute many positive studies. Ask yourself, which is more likely correct, many studies that agree, or one that disagrees?

RESEARCH STUDY QUESTIONS

When you read about a contradictory medical study, ask yourself these questions before blindly accepting it.

1. Is it a meta-analysis instead of a real clinical study?
2. Were the doses used too small to do any good?
3. Were the doses used much higher than any human would ever take?
4. Was the studied substance natural or synthetic?
5. Was there anything radically different from previous studies so that an apples-to-apples comparison cannot be made?
6. Was the study commissioned by a drug company to discredit natural alternatives to one of their drugs?
7. Was it done in vitro (test tube) or in vivo (living animal)?
8. Were human trials conducted or just animal experiments?

In vitro or in vivo animal studies are necessary before human trials can begin. They should not be dismissed, but rather regarded with caution. Human trials may show different results.

An article in the *Chicago Tribune* (July 28, 2005) said that taking Echinacea (purple coneflower) to ward off colds or reduce its symptoms was ineffective according to a large study. Unfortunately, the reporters never asked the researchers detailed questions to determine if the study was valid.

If I was one of the reporters, I would have asked these questions:

1. What species of Echinacea did you use? Was it the same used in other studies and by those reporting good results?
2. What part of the plant did you use? Was it the root, stem, flower, or the whole plant? How does that

compare to other studies and by those reporting good results?

3. Did you use a standardized extract of the active ingredients? Was it the same used in other studies and by those reporting good results?
4. What dose did you use? Was it the same used in other studies and by those reporting good results?
5. You used only the rhinovirus type 39 to induce colds. What about other viruses and bacteria? What if the infection was not concentrated in the nose?

The New York Times (July 28, 2005) also reported that one of the authors, Dr. Rudolf Bauer, said that the study should be repeated with other Echinacea species, preparations and doses. Maybe he knew that the study was flawed – and it was. The study did not use the same commercial grade Echinacea found in health food stores and the dose was too low (330 mg vs. 3 grams required).

The point I am trying to make is do not blindly accept what the media reports as fact. Check it out yourself. Ask detailed, intelligent questions before you decide.

DISCLAIMER

Please read the disclaimer in the front of the book. You and your physician should work together as a team; therefore, it is important to have a health care provider who is open to alternative medicine instead of relying solely on prescription drugs and evasive procedures. In some cases, you may need to change physicians.

Now it is time to meet the enemies. In the next chapter you will learn about some of the "bad" guys in your body that can cause miserable allergy and asthma problems. We must understand our internal enemies before we can hope to defeat them.

CHAPTER 2

MEET THE ENEMY

The human body is extremely complex. When everything works as it is supposed to, we enjoy good health. Unfortunately, things go wrong. The same immune system that protects us from illness can go awry and produce allergies and asthma. Both of these conditions result from a severe inflammatory response to various stimuli or irritants.

You are probably familiar with one of the culprits – histamine. Prescription and OTC anti-histamine drugs are widely used to alleviate allergy symptoms. In many cases, they don't do a very good job. Why? Histamine is only one of the chemicals involved in allergic and asthmatic responses. Look at this abbreviated list of culprits: [8]

Inflammatory Cytokines (Interleukins)

IL-1 beta

IL- 2

IL-4

IL-5

IL-8

Immune Response Cells

Eosinophils cause bronchial constriction in asthma

Neutrophils destroy tissue if overactive

T cells are responsible for hypersensitivity reactions

Mast cells release histamine and leukotrienes

Basophils release histamine and other chemicals

Polymorphonuclear leukocytes

Chemical Attractors

Histamine causes contraction of bronchial smooth muscles

Eotaxin

Other Inflammatory Substances

Leukotrienes cause inflammation and bronchial constriction

Prostaglandin E2 causes inflammation

Nitric Oxide causes inflammation

Don't let these big words scare you. I merely want to make the point that histamine is only one part of the problem and it is not near the root cause. When you deal with histamine, the inflammatory process is already roaring full speed ahead.

Only controlling histamine is akin to having a water main break and pumping the never-ending flow of water into a lake instead of fixing the root cause, a broken water pipe. Most drugs do not act on the root causes, but merely ameliorate symptoms. The body continues to be damaged by the underlying disease, as well as by the side effects of the drugs themselves.

The interleukins, for example, are cell-signaling chemicals (cytokines) that are very close to the beginning of the allergy immune response. They control the immune response to a high degree. We must control the "controllers" if we are to successfully manage allergies and asthma.

You will see many of these chemicals mentioned later in the book. There is an arsenal of various herbal extracts and vitamins that can counteract the uncontrolled inflammatory response that they produce. You will also learn about new weapons that you can use in your fight against allergies and asthma.

Immune Response Cells

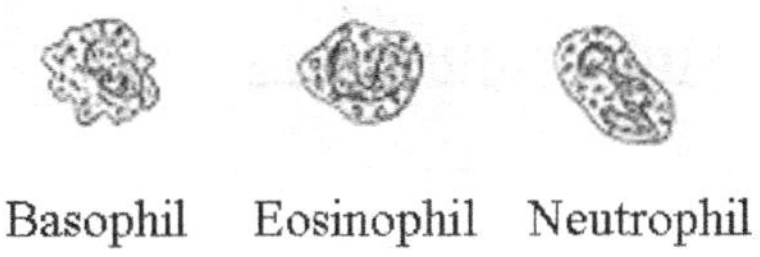

Figure 1. Immune Response Cells

THE IMMUNE RESPONSE

Now for those of you who want to learn a little about how all these substances fit together (or want to impress your doctor), here is a brief scenario. In a TYPE I immune reaction, a foreign substance called an antigen or allergen enters the body and binds with a mast cell or basophil. Attached to a mast cell or basophil is an antibody called immunoglobulin (IgE). Each IgE antibody is designed to work with only one antigen.[1]

The IgE antibody controls the mast cell, waiting for the correct antigen to activate it. If the correct antigen attaches itself, the mast cell spews out histamine, leukotrienes and cytokines (cell-signaling chemicals). These chemicals cause inflammation and bronchial constriction.[1]

Some of these substances, such as IgE and leukotrienes, are over expressed in allergy and asthma patients. A normal body defensive reaction can turn ugly because of this over-expression. An IgE allergic reaction can be due to pollen, mold, dust mites, insect stings, animal dander, or certain foods.[1]

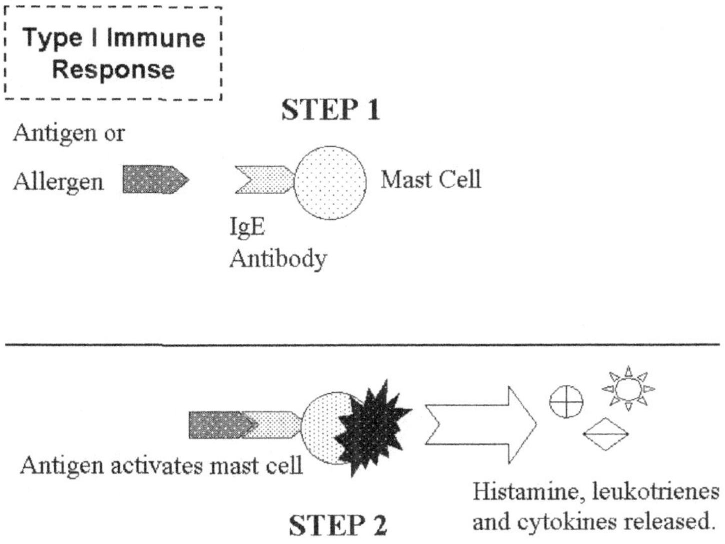

Figure 2. Immune Response

ALLERGIES

Allergic rhinitis (upper-airway allergies) basically starts with inflammatory cytokines IL-1 beta, IL-2, IL-4, IL-5 and IL-8 activating and proliferating immune response cells such as eosinophils, neutrophils and T cells. These cells collect rapidly in the blood and nasal fluids. Histamine and eotaxin attract eosinophils into the nasal passages and airways.[2, 8]

The result is a massive collection of cells that impedes the flow of air to the lungs. It also causes the familiar nasal congestion and swelling.

Anti-histamines help by inhibiting the release of histamine from mast cells. They do not, however, decrease neutrophil or T cell activation or proliferation. This is an extremely important fact. The root causes still exist! [3, 8]

The high levels of these cells can cause free radical damage to normal tissues. The stage is set for lung damage and possibly heart disease. Lungs that are continually inflamed can be permanently damaged.

I am not aware of any prescription or OTC drugs that address this underlying, dangerous situation. Taking drugs long-term or indefinitely is not the answer. They may create other serious conditions. Later in this book, I will show you how to attack the cell proliferation problem by natural means.

ALLERGY-INDUCED ASTHMA

Asthma can be induced by an allergic reaction. Asthma patients have an overactive antibody immune system. This immune system is controlled by cytokines. Cytokines signal the on-off activity of mast cells, basophils, eosinophils and B cells.

The suspected link between allergic rhinitis and asthma is a high eosinophil count in nasal mucous. Many people suffer from both seasonal allergies and asthma. In those people, eosinophils are the most important factor in predicting upper-airway and lower-airway function.[4, 5, 9]

Researchers were able to duplicate the smooth muscle thickening in asthmatics by repeatedly exposing rats to allergens. They observed a large increase in the number of T cells, eosinophils, lymphocytes and neutrophils in the lung fluid. These cells are drawn into the lung tissue by histamine and other chemical attractors. The belief is that lung tissue is scarred by free radical damage caused by these cells.[6, 9] Allergy control, therefore, is critical in preventing lung tissue damage.

Asthma Airway Obstruction

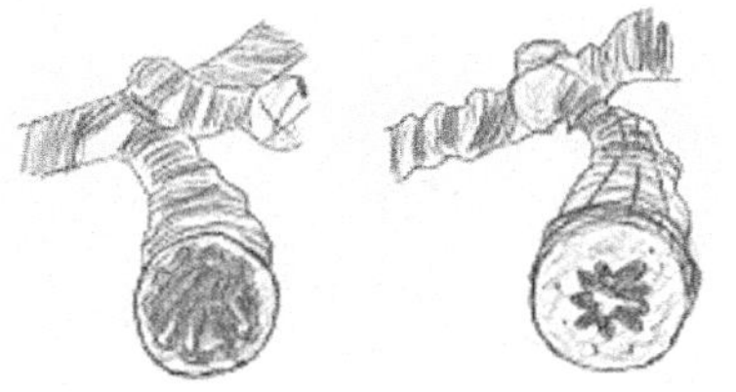

Figure 3. Asthma Airway Obstruction Of Bronchiole

EXERCISE-INDUCED ASTHMA

There is also exercise-induced asthma. Its cause is unknown, but two mainstream theories exist.

The *Water Loss Theory* states that during exercise, air is inhaled through the mouth instead of the nose. Consequently, the air that reaches the lungs is colder and dryer than if it had been inhaled through the nose. The lungs make up for the dryness by contributing their own water vapor. This dries the airway and causes various physiological changes. One of the changes (hyper-osmolarity) is believed to cause the release of histamine, leukotrienes and prostaglandins.[7]

In the *Heat-exchange Theory*, increased air intake during exercise cools the airways. After exercise, a re-warming process begins that can narrow the airway through a complex series of events causing bronchial spasms and the release of inflammatory chemicals.[7]

In the next chapters we will meet the “good guys”. You will discover an arsenal of natural herbal extracts, vitamins and minerals that can combat the powerful inflammatory chemicals and cell proliferation that cause allergies and asthma. Your arsenal will include several super weapons as well as numerous support troops.

CHAPTER 3

THE NATURAL ARSENAL PART I

Now we are ready to look at the arsenal of natural weapons in the fight against allergies and asthma. Three super weapons will be unveiled in a later chapter. But first, the conventional support troops.

Support troops are the foundation of good health. Our bodies need adequate amounts of vitamins and minerals each day; in addition, we need protein (to make amino acids), carbohydrates and fat (lipids) for energy, defense and body repair. You cannot expect good health without a good foundation. Even if you use one of the super weapons mentioned later in the book, you still need to give your body the basic support that it needs.

If you ignore this chapter, you will greatly diminish your chances for a normal, healthy life. You will also decrease the effects of the "big guns". Just as a real army must work together in a coordinated effort in order to be victorious, your body's support and assault troops must work together as a team to win the victory over disease.

DEFINITIONS

You will see certain abbreviations in the following sections. In case you've wondered what terms like "mg" mean, here are the definitions.

mg = milligram = $^{1}/_{1,000}$ gram

mcg = microgram = $^{1}/_{1,000,000}$ gram

IU = International Unit

MULTI-VITAMINS AND MINERALS

Multi-vitamin and mineral supplements (herein referred to as MVM) are familiar to most people. You can buy them at your local grocery store – if you want to waste your money. What is wrong with many MVM supplements?

First, you are probably getting the bare minimum dose of many vitamins. Some MVM's do not even have 100% of the Daily Value (DV). The DV's are much too small in most cases. So, the first problem is the ridiculously low doses of many vitamins and minerals.

The 100% DV of vitamin C, for example, is 60 mg. That amount of vitamin C is the bare minimum needed to prevent scurvy in a healthy individual. It is not the maximum amount you should take, nor is it the amount for optimum health. Remember, the DV also assumes that a person is healthy. Some 100 % DV amounts may be acceptable, such as vitamin D 400 IU, biotin 300 mcg, iodine 150 mcg, zinc 15 mg, folate 400 mcg and copper 2 mg. Most B vitamins, however, should be in the 25 to 50 mg range.

Why should some of the dosages be so much higher than 100% of the DV? If, for example, you take 25 mg of vitamin B-1, your intake will be 1667% higher than the recommended Daily Value. The famous nutrition researcher, Bruce Ames, provides the answer.

He and his colleagues state that for many people the Recommended Daily Allowance (RDA) is not sufficient to avoid major illness and death. Ames reported that approximately 50 human genetic diseases could be corrected or lessened by taking high doses of nutrients. Vitamins and minerals activate the enzymes in our bodies that are necessary for life. Defective enzymes cause genetic diseases. [1]

The high doses help restore defective enzyme activity responsible for these genetic diseases. Ames reported that many people were saved from death or crippling disease by consuming 10 to 500 times the RDA.[1]

Another MVM problem may be the total absence of substances like choline, inositol, selenium, pantothenic acid and chromium.

A third issue is the form of the vitamins and minerals. Some forms are not easily absorbed and usable by the body (bio-available). Minerals should be chelated (combined with an organic substance for absorption); otherwise, you are swallowing a literal rock. Your body doesn't absorb rock very well. Two absorbable examples are ChromMate® for chromium and L-Selenomethionine for selenium.

Avoid tablets whenever possible. A tablet may pass right through your body without much of it ever being absorbed. Some nurses call them "bullets". Make sure your MVM is in capsule form.

There is one more thing to consider in choosing an MVM. Some MVM manufacturers add a nutrient that has had some national publicity in order to get you to buy. The problem is that the amount that they add is worthless!

Take the nutrient lutein, which studies show can help with eye diseases such as macular degeneration. If the bottle touts 500 mcg (millionths of a gram) of lutein, should you be impressed? Absolutely not! Research studies indicate that you need 15 – 20 mg (thousandths of a gram) of lutein per day. That MVM would have <u>30 times too little</u> lutein to do any good. Don't waste your money on MVM's like that. Your only defense is to be well informed.

The MVM is the shotgun in your arsenal. It covers a broad area with one shot. It provides the cornerstone of your nutrient foundation. Many of the supplements listed hereafter are also found in your MVM. Be sure to add up the amounts you get per day from all sources.

◙ An MVM should have at least these typical amounts:

Vitamin A (at least $^{2}/_{3}$ as beta-carotene) 15,000 IU

Vitamin D 400 IU

Vitamin B-1 25 mg

Vitamin B-2 25 mg

Vitamin B-3 (niacinamide)

Vitamin B-6 25 mg

Vitamin B-12 100 mcg

Biotin 300 mcg

Folate (folic acid) 400 mcg

Vitamin B-5 (pantothenic acid) 50 – 100 mg

Iodine 150 mcg

Zinc 15 mg

Selenium 200 mcg

Copper 1 – 2 mg

Manganese 5 mg

Chromium (polynicotinate) 200 mcg

Molybdenum 150 mcg

Choline 25 mg +

Inositol 25 mg +

Potassium 99 mg

Calcium (800 – 1000 mg with additional supplements)

Magnesium (400 – 750 mg with additional supplements)

VITAMIN A (BETA-CAROTENE)

Vitamin A is essential for healthy lung tissue. Beta-carotene is a precursor to vitamin A. It is converted to vitamin A by the body as needed. Beta-carotene is also an antioxidant that protects against free radical damage. Free radicals are produced by many chemical reactions in the body and by diseases. Free radicals are dangerous because they can attack normal molecules. If they attack DNA molecules, mutations may occur and the stage is set for diseases such as cancer.

Researchers in Israel reported that 64 mg of beta-carotene per day protected over 50% of a group of asthmatic patients who had attacks resulting from exercise. Their theory is that exercise causes free-radical damage and beta-carotene helps because it is an antioxidant. More research is needed to determine if this is true.[2]

Note that 1 mg of beta-carotene = 1,667 IU of beta-carotene. The study cited, therefore, used (64 X 1667) 106,688 IU of beta-carotene. That is an extremely high dose and is not recommended without physician supervision.

▼ *Beta-carotene Cautions*

Do not take large doses of beta-carotene if you have liver disease. Taking large doses of regular vitamin A (retinal) for a long period of time may cause liver damage.

◘ Recommended beta-carotene dose is 5000 – 20,000 IU per day taken with some fat. Beta-carotene should be in your MVM.

VITAMIN B-6

Asthma sufferers have lower blood levels of vitamin B-6. Supplementation with vitamin B-6 may alleviate symptoms in some asthmatics.

In a two-month double-blind trial, researchers found that 200 mg of vitamin B-6 reduced the severity of asthma in children. They were also able to reduce their medication.[3]

Another study showed that adults had a significant decrease in the frequency and severity of asthma attacks when they took 50 mg of vitamin B-6 twice a day.[4]

Not everyone is helped by vitamin B-6. One double-blind study found that even high amounts of vitamin B-6 did not help asthma patients who required steroid drugs.[5]

◘ B-6 dose is 50 – 100 mg per day. Vitamin B-6 should be in your MVM.

VITAMIN B-12

Some people suffer an asthma attack when they eat foods containing sulfite food additives. One study showed that vitamin B-12 may help reduce symptoms in such people. The study used the common cyanocobalamin form of vitamin B-12.[6]

A much better form of B-12 is methylcobalamin. Cyanocobalamin has to be converted to methylcobalamin in the liver. A superior way is to dissolve methylcobalamin lozenges under the tongue. Methylcobalamin does not have to be processed by the liver and goes directly into the blood stream where it can be used immediately.

Lack of B-12 is a serious problem. Vitamin B-12 changes folate (another B vitamin) into its active form. Lack of activated folate will cause anemia. There is no B-12 in a purely vegetarian diet. Vitamin B-12 is found in meats, eggs and dairy products.

▼ ***Vitamin B-12 Cautions***

Do not take more than 4000 mcg (4mg) without physician supervision.

◙ Recommended dose is 500 – 2000 mcg of methyl-cobalamin per day.

VITAMIN C

Vitamin C is a natural, antihistamine and antioxidant. It helps prevent histamine from being released and mops up excess histamine in the blood. One large study showed that young children with asthma experienced less wheezing if they ate a diet rich in fruit containing vitamin C.[7]

Taking 1000 mg (1 gram) of vitamin C per day decreases bronchial spasms according to one double-blind study.[8, 9]

Another double-blind study found that 1000 mg of vitamin C per day, for 14 weeks, reduced both the severity and frequency of asthma attacks for Nigerian adult asthmatics.[10]

◙ Take between 1000 and 4500 mg of Ester-C™ spread out over the day. Ester-C™ is non-acidic and will not give you an upset stomach. Ascorbic acid vitamin C will. The Ester-C™ should include a bioflavonoid complex.

VITAMIN E

Vitamin E is a family of fat-soluble compounds that possess anti-oxidant capabilities. The family has two main branches: tocopherol and tocotrienol. Each branch, in turn, has alpha, beta, delta and gamma compounds.

Most vitamin E products consist of d-alpha tocopherol acetate or d-alpha tocopherol succinate. Never take dl-alpha tocopherol. It is a synthetic version. You want natural, mixed tocopherols for maximum effect. A "dl-" means synthetic and the prefix "d-" means organic. If possible, use natural vitamin E that contains the whole family of alpha, beta, delta and gamma compounds.

So, how does vitamin E help us in our fight against asthma and allergies? You may recall that leukotrienes cause inflammation and airway constriction. Tocopherol and tocopherol acetate inhibit the formation of leukotrienes.[11, 22]

In addition, lower blood concentrations of IgE and less allergen sensitivity are found with higher levels of vitamin E intake.[12, 22] IgE initiates an immune response when an allergen attaches itself. Decrease the number IgE antibodies and you decrease the possibility for an allergic reaction. Therefore, taking vitamin E may lessen the possibility of an allergic reaction in the first place.

▼ ***Vitamin E Cautions***

Consult your doctor before taking vitamin E if you are taking anti-coagulant medication. Do not take more than 800 IU per day. If you have high blood pressure, you should start off with 100 IU and gradually build up to 400 – 800 IU per day.

◙ Vitamin E dose is 400 – 800 IU per day of natural, mixed tocopherols or d-alpha tocopherol.[23] Some of your vitamin E dose should be in your MVM.

MAGNESIUM

Over 300 chemical reactions in the human body involve magnesium. Asthmatics usually have low levels of magnesium.[13] Intravenous treatment with magnesium can halt an acute asthma attack.[14] But what about oral intake of magnesium?

One double-blind study found that taking 400 mg per day for 3 weeks significantly improved symptoms, but did not change airflow measurements.[15] Additional studies have also shown this result.[16]

One important study involved 89 children aged 4 to 16 years with mild to moderate asthma. When given 290 mg of magnesium citrate per day for 12 weeks, bronchodilator use was significantly lower than when they took a placebo. The researchers suggested that magnesium supplementation provides a benefit in mild to moderate asthmatic children.[17] Oral magnesium use in severe asthma cases has not been well documented.

Magnesium supplementation appears to improve symptoms without improving objective airflow parameters. In other words, magnesium does not appear to heal already damaged lung and bronchial tissue. Doctors may dismiss the value of magnesium because they don't see a measurable difference on airflow tests, but let us not lose sight of the fact that symptoms eased and bronchodilator use decreased by taking magnesium orally. Those are two positive benefits from an inexpensive mineral that we all should be taking anyway.

Also consider magnesium for its many other health benefits that are beyond the scope of this book. Definitely include it in your arsenal.

Magnesium should be taken separately from calcium because calcium inhibits its absorption. If you must take them together, keep the calcium to magnesium ratio close to 1:1 to help absorption.

▼ *Magnesium Cautions*

Consult your doctor before taking magnesium if you have kidney (renal) problems.

◘ Dose to alleviate asthmatic symptoms is 400 – 750 mg per day. Use chelated magnesium for better absorption. Magnesium oxide, by itself, is poorly absorbed. Other good forms include magnesium citrate, aspartate, succinate and taurinate.

SELENIUM

Low levels of selenium constitute a high risk for asthma.[18, 19, 20, 21] Selenium may have a protective effect because of its anti-oxidant properties. In a small trial of 11 patients, six showed clinical improvement when given 100 mcg of sodium selenite per day for 14 weeks.[24] Only one of ten in the placebo group showed improvement. Better results may have been obtained with the now recommended 200 mcg of selenium in more easily absorbed forms than sodium selenite.

◙ Get 200 mcg of selenium each day. It's important for the prevention of certain cancers, too. Selenium should be in your MVM.

CHAPTER 4

THE NATURAL ARSENAL PART II

The last chapter dealt with vitamins, minerals and the multi-vitamin-mineral (MVM) supplement. In Part II we will continue adding to our arsenal. We will cover special supplements and certain herbal extracts. ALWAYS start with the MINIMUM dose for an herbal supplement just in case you are allergic to the plant!

After three days, increase your dose gradually to be safe. Most people are not allergic to the herbs listed below, but they can be checked against any allergy tests that you may have had. Now prepare to load up the next round.

BOSWELLIA

We need a little background before discussing Boswellia. Here's the unfortunate sequence of events:

1. The body makes arachidonic acid from linoleic acid, an omega-6 fatty acid.
2. 5-Lox converts arachidonic acid into highly inflammatory leukotrienes we learned about earlier; therefore, 5-Lox is one of the bad guys we have to control.[1]

The East Indian herb frankincense, called Boswellia serrata, does inhibit 5-Lox.[2] Remember frankincense in the Christmas story? The wise men gave frankincense to the Christ-child. Frankincense was highly valued because of its medicinal properties. You can use Boswellia extracts in your fight against asthma. It effectively inhibits the leukotriene B4, which causes inflammation, free radical damage and adhesion of inflammatory cells.[2]

By the way, also take Boswellia every time that you use an NSAID (non-steroidal anti-inflammatory drug). An NSAID, such as ibuprofen, actually activates 5-Lox. So while the NSAID inhibits the COX-2 inflammatory pathway, it also generates inflammation through the 5-Lox pathway.[19] The latter can destroy cartilage and cause wheezing. That is why an NSAID should not be taken for more than three consecutive days. Take your NSAID with Boswellia to help limit the 5-Lox inflammation and save your cartilage.

◙ Take three, 300 mg capsules of Boswellia per day. Make sure it's standardized to contain at least 65% boswellic acids. Cut the dose in half for children.

COENZYME Q10 (COQ10)

I mentioned CoQ10 in the preface. It is a familiar friend. It can help with many different diseases, including allergies. Just what does CoQ10 do? It helps produce ATP (adenosine triphosphate), which is the energy source for your cells. Without CoQ10 you would have no energy (ATP) for life and you would die.[17]

CoQ10 is also a special antioxidant that is able to reach the mitochondrial membrane. The mitochondria produce energy for the cells. [17] Many diseases, such as congestive heart failure and cancer, deplete CoQ10 levels. Surprisingly, a study showed that 14 out of 36 patients with allergy conditions had CoQ10 levels equal to a group of gravely ill cardiac patients (Ye et al. 1988). That's reason enough to supplement with CoQ10.[17]

◘ Take 60 – 300 mg of CoQ10 each day to get your levels back up.

FISH OIL

The verdict is still out on fish oil. Some studies indicate that fish oil does not help asthmatics.[3] The negative results, however, may be due to several factors.

1. First, the studies may not have lasted long enough.
2. Users may not have taken enough vitamin E with the fish oil to prevent it from turning rancid in the body, thus, producing a negative effect instead of a positive one.
3. The amount of the DHA component may have been too small to do any good. DHA may be more responsible for many of the good effects of fish oil than EPA.

On the positive side, some fish oil studies show partial relief from allergens that can trigger asthma attacks.[4, 5] Children who eat oily fish may have a lower risk of developing asthma.[6] In a double-blind study, children were given 84 mg of EPA and 36 mg of DHA per day. Exposure to food and environmental allergens were strictly controlled. The fish oil consumption resulted in significant improvement of asthma symptoms.[7]

Please note that 36 mg of DHA is very low. Better results may have been obtained with higher DHA and lower EPA amounts. Nevertheless, fish oil should be considered, at least for children. Be sure to read the cautions below.

▼ *Fish Oil Cautions*

The main active ingredients in fish oil are EPA and DHA. DHA oxidizes easily in the body, which means that it can produce numerous unwanted free radicals. The simple solution is to always take fish oil with sufficient vitamin E. Vitamin E will mop up those free radicals, allowing you to reap the benefits of fish oil.

One more thing – if you do take fish oil, **make sure it is molecularly distilled to remove heavy metal contamination such as mercury.** Fish are routinely contaminated with this deadly poison.

◘ Take 1500 –3000 mg per day of molecularly distilled fish oil that is high in DHA. Take it with your with vitamin E.

LYCOPENE

The tomato antioxidant, lycopene, can help reduce asthma symptoms induced by exercise. In a double-blind trial, 55% of the participants had significantly reduced exercise-induced asthma symptoms after taking 30 mg of lycopene for one week. When they took a placebo instead, the amount of air that they could blow out was reduced more than 15% after 7 minutes of exercise.[8, 18] Lycopene costs very little to try and the odds are in your favor.

◘ Take 20 – 30 mg of lycopene each day with vitamin C to enhance its effect.

N-ACETYL-CYSTEINE (NAC)

Before we discuss NAC, we need to learn about the body's master antioxidant, glutathione. Glutathione (GSH) is made in the body from glutamic acid, cysteine and glycine.[17] Glutathione protects the body against free radicals and detoxifies such drugs as Tylenol®. We cannot survive without glutathione.

What is the connection between glutathione and allergies and asthma? Let's review a little. Interleukin 4 (IL-4) is involved in the production of IgE antibodies. IgE is over expressed in people suffering from allergies or asthma. This over-expression causes severe reactions. Lowering IL-4 should lower IgE production, which, in turn, should reduce allergy and asthma problems.

A 2001 study showed that supplementation with NAC and glutathione lowered levels of IL-4 and enhanced T-cell proliferation.[9, 17] NAC has also been used to treat bronchitis and other lung ailments because of its ability to thin mucous (expectorant).

NAC is a precursor to glutathione. The body can convert NAC into glutathione.[17] Glutathione is an expensive supplement, but NAC is inexpensive. NAC is also absorbed well and not oxidized when taken with vitamin C. NAC is, therefore, the supplement of choice to increase glutathione levels. Other supplements that raise glutathione levels are alpha lipoic acid, Pycnogenol®, bilberry and turmeric.

◙ Take 600 – 1800 mg of NAC per day with 1000 mg of vitamin C for every 600 mg of NAC. [17] Also take it with selenium from your MVM.

PYCNOGENOL®

Pycnogenol® is a standardized extract from the French maritime pine bark that grows in the southwestern part of France. The researcher, Rohdewald, states that it helps in three ways: [10, 18]

1. Reduces asthma symptoms
2. Reduces circulating leukotrienes
3. Improves lung function in asthmatics

◙ Dose is 100 mg daily of standardized Pycnogenol®. Unfortunately, it is relatively expensive.

QUERCETIN

Quercetin is a bioflavonoid found in onions, apples, broccoli, black tea and other foods.[11, 12] Research has found that quercetin can strongly inhibit the release of histamine from basophils and mast cells.[13, 14, 15, 16]

Middleton and others report that quercetin is able to stabilize cell membranes, which prevents histamine from pouring out into the bloodstream. Quercetin also helps inhibit the enzymes phospholipase A2 and lipoxygenase. Those enzymes help make leukotrienes from arachidonic acid.[14]

We already know that leukotrienes are big contributors to the misery of allergies and asthma. So you can see that quercetin helps us in two important ways.

Quercetin products are sold many times in conjunction with bromelain, another anti-inflammatory supplement. I do not recommend this combination because bromelain can cause heart palpitations. Quercetin combined with vitamin C is ideal.

▼ ***Quercetin Cautions***

Find a bromelain-free capsule of quercetin. Bromelain can cause heart palpitations in some people.

◙ Dose is 200 – 400 mg, 3 times a day. Take with vitamin C.

SUPPORT ARSENAL CONCLUSION

You may obtain your arsenal products from *Vitacost* (www.vitacost.com) and *Swanson Health Products* (www.swansonvitamins.com). I have no connection or financial interest in any company listed in this book. I am merely providing the information to save you research time.

Now it is time to roll out the big guns to use with your support arsenal. Here come the super weapons!

CHAPTER 5

SUPER, NATURAL WEAPONS

Next, we roll out our super weapon to attack the neutrophil and T cell proliferation problem mentioned in chapter 2. As you may recall, current drugs DO NOT address this critical problem. They may reduce histamine or leukotrienes, but they do not reduce the large number of activated neutrophils and T cells that are free to cause continuous tissue damage.

But Rosmarinic Acid Extract can!

ROSMARINC ACID EXTRACT

Rosmarinic acid is a polyphenol found in rosemary, perilla leaf, basil, mint and sage. Human studies have found that rosmarinic acid can suppress allergic reactions.[1, 12, 13] Rosmarinic acid works by preventing the activation of immune response cells (see chapter 2) and by inducing cellular suicide, called apoptosis, in already activated immune response cells.[2, 3, 12, 13] This powerful supplement works on two fronts – inhibiting the activation of T cells that cause severe reactions and preventing their proliferation.

The important difference between rosmarinic acid and drugs is that **Rosmarinic acid helps eliminate the underlying cause of tissue damage by destroying excess immune response cells that have been activated by an allergic response.** The non-activated neutrophils and T cells are not affected and are ready to fight off true infections.[4, 13]

Rosmarinic acid is truly a remarkable substance in our arsenal.

In one study, researchers showed that rosmarinic acid taken orally strongly reduced IL-beta, IL-8 and nitric oxide. Remember the first two culprits from chapter 2? They are cytokines that signal inflammation. IL-8 is believed to be largely responsible for acute lung injury by causing neutrophils to accumulate in the lungs. That makes rosmarinic acid very important in the fight against asthma.[4, 13]

Another study found that rosmarinic acid inhibited the IL-2 activation of T cells. It also showed that rosmarinic acid disposes of excess activated T cells by inducing cellular suicide. The killing process took about 24 hours.[5, 13]

The final research study presented here shows great hope for seasonal allergy sufferers. Patients were given a total daily, rosmarinic acid dose of 50 mg or 200 mg. By day 3, both groups taking rosmarinic acid showed significantly reduced amounts of polymorphonuclear leukocytes and neutrophils in their nasal fluid as compared to the control group.[1, 12, 13]

The researchers concluded that the inhibiting of polymorphonuclear leukocytes infiltration into the nostrils is partly responsible for alleviating the symptoms of allergic rhinitis. Rosmarinic acid did an especially good job of relieving eye-related symptoms. No side effects were observed. Blood cell counts, hepatic and renal tests showed rosmarinic acid to be safe.[1, 6, 12, 13, 14]

You can see that rosmarinic acid can attack many of the culprits on our list of enemies in chapter 2. It is a safe and effective treatment of seasonal allergies. It truly is a super weapon in our arsenal of natural supplements.

◙ Dose for rosmarinic acid extract is 100 mg one or two times daily after breakfast. See the dose section under luteolin for a source of both rosmarinic acid and luteolin.

LUTEOLIN

Luteolin is another plant flavonoid. It is also found in the perilla plant along with rosmarinic acid. The Japanese have used luteolin in herbal formulations for centuries to treat bronchial asthma.[7, 14] A study by the Osaka University Medical School found that luteolin was the most powerful inhibitor of IL-4 production by human basophils and T cells. IL-4 and IL-5 are potent allergic initiators.[8, 14]

Luteolin taken orally also inhibits IL-5. IL-5 promotes the proliferation of eosinophils. Eosinophils, you may recall, collect in the airways and nasal passages during an allergy attack. They cause swelling and air restriction.[9, 14]

In rat experiments, luteolin also inhibited the release of histamine from mast cells when the rats were exposed to IgE antibodies.[10] Luteolin is a great weapon in our arsenal because it has tremendous anti-inflammatory and anti-allergic activity in living organisms.[11, 14]

I know that this is quite difficult to digest, so I've included a diagram which summarizes where luteolin and rosmarinic acid inhibit the various asthma and allergy producing chemicals. Start at the bottom of the diagram and work your way up to high-level symptoms.

Notice that luteolin and rosmarinic acid block the early stages of allergy and asthma attacks. They don't just inhibit histamine like OTC drugs do, but rather attack many other powerful chemicals involved in the vicious process.

You may recall from chapter two, that the suspected link between allergic rhinitis and asthma is a high eosinophil count in nasal mucous. The diagram clearly shows that luteolin inhibits IL-5, which, in turn, causes the increase in eosinophils. Luteolin, therefore, is extremely important in preventing asthma from developing in the first place.

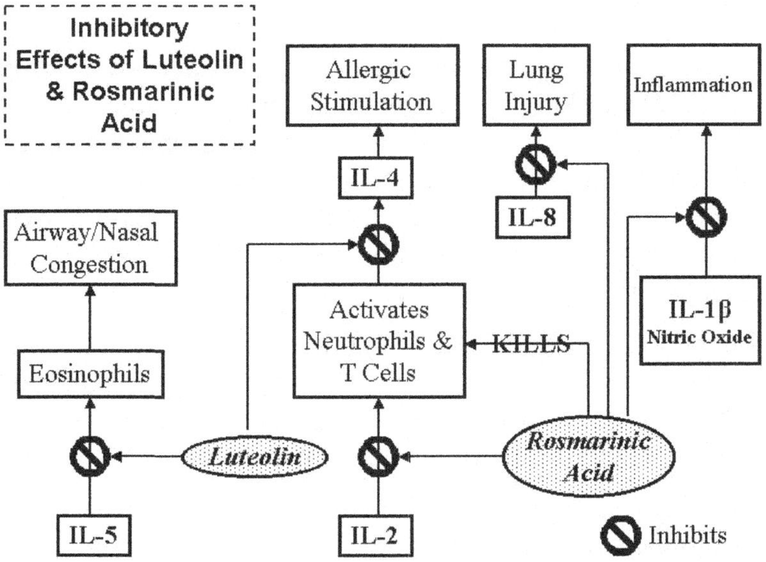

Figure 4. Luteolin and Rosmarinic Acid Effects

◘ Dose for luteolin extract is 4 mg one or two times daily after breakfast.

A good source of both rosmarinic acid and luteolin is found in **ROSMARINIC ACID EXTRACT** from **LIFE EXTENSION™** (www.lef.org). Follow the instructions on the bottle. You may save a buck or two if you search the web for other companies that carry this particular product. Again, I have no connection or financial interest in any company listed in this book. I am merely providing the information as a convenience.

YAMOA™

I have included Yamoa even though it does not have scientific evidence at the present time to support its use. There has to be considerable supplement use and anecdotal evidence before science becomes interested. People used the supplements discussed earlier long before actual scientific studies were conducted. Yamoa is in that category now. I've included it because it may have considerable promise.

No one claims that it can cure asthma or allergies, but a certain percentage of users have, indeed, reported cures. Children over one year old can use it, too.

Just what is Yamoa? Yamoa is derived from the bark of the Funtumia Elastica gum tree, but is actually named after Jerry Yamoa who brought it to the UK from Ghana. His grandmother, Akua Asirifia, had used this herb to treat asthma and hay fever back in Ghana.[15]

Jerry Yamoa was a postal worker in South London and had seen many of his colleagues suffering from asthma and hay fever. He gave the herb to them to see if it would help. The results were very encouraging.[15]

Since the small, unscientific trial in South London, the success of Yamoa spread. It was reported in national newspapers such as the Daily Mail and featured on the London Today TV program. Clinical trials are now being designed.[15]

Yamoa is apparently useful in conditions such as asthma, hay fever, bronchitis and sinusitis. What makes Yamoa unique is that many people report lasting benefits after the full dose has been completed. Some have even reported complete symptomatic relief after consuming only one container of Yamoa powder or vegetarian capsules. This lasting effect occurs in one or two months, and in some cases in only a few days! [15]

Of course, it does not work for everyone. The company asks users to submit their experience with Yamoa, so that they can determine its effectiveness for different types of people and conditions.

Here are the results of what Yamoa users have said as of the writing of this book, according to the Yamoa brochure. The reported conditions include hay fever and asthma.[15]

Question: How long did you take Yamoa powder for?

One month: 67%

Two months: 8%

Three months: 17%

Four months: 8%

More: 0%

Question: How long was it before you noticed a change in your condition?

Within a couple days: 8%

Within a week or two: 34%

Within a month: 33%

Longer than a month: 17%

Longer than four months: 8%

Question: How were you affected by Yamoa powder?

Total symptomatic relief: 17%

Marked improvement: 34%

Mild improvement: 33%

It only worked while I took it: 8%

It didn't work for me: 8%

For asthmatics, the average peak flow rate reading before Yamoa treatment was 350. After completing the total Yamoa dose it increased an average of 70 points to 420. The group reported 78 asthma attacks per year before taking Yamoa and 22 attacks per year after taking Yamoa.[15]

Yamoa is another super weapon to consider. It is relatively expensive, but it may be worthwhile if you happen to get total relief with one container. You'll have to do the cost-benefit-risk analysis. Safety does not appear to be a concern based on the user comments.

▼ ***Yamoa Cautions***

Check their web site before ordering. The only reaction listed was from one lady on 0.5 mg of Norvasc blood pressure medication. The reaction ceased when she stopped taking Yamoa.[15]

◙ Follow the instructions that come with Yamoa. If at all possible, use the capsules instead of the powder. Adults take 1 – 2 capsules per day. One bottle contains 60 vegetarian capsules.

Read their web site thoroughly before ordering (www.yamoapowder.com).

UK Phone: + 44 1865 355515

UK Fax: +44 (0) 1865 311434

SUMMARY

You now have a complete arsenal to combat both allergies and asthma. Many supplements are supportive of the super weapons and should not be belittled. The following figure shows the building block effect of the supplements with vitamins and minerals forming the foundation of the pyramid.

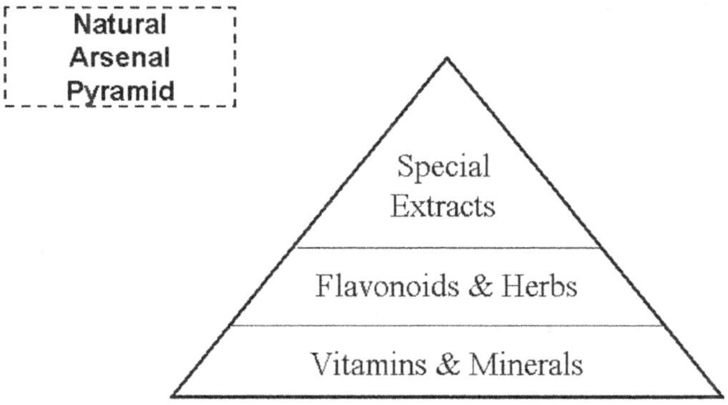

Figure 5. Natural Arsenal Pyramid

CHAPTER 6

GARBAGE IN, DISEASE OUT

There is an old saying, "You are what you eat". Today we could also add "You are what you breathe". Your health depends on what you eat and breathe. No, I am not going to lecture you about eating more fruits and veggies and less fat. Neither am I advocating one diet over another. This chapter will examine what has happened to our food supplies. We will also look at ozone and air purifier products. Are some products actually dangerous to your health?

Have you ever wondered why there has been a dramatic increase in diabetes, heart disease, asthma, allergies and cancer? Asthma has increased tremendously in the past few years. It is estimated that 12 to 14 million Americans have asthma. More than 4 million of them are under 18 years of age.[1]

Perhaps we should look at the food we eat and the air we breathe. If we put garbage into our bodies, we can expect a bad outcome, namely, disease.

OZONE AND ASTHMA

Oxygen, which is necessary for human life, consists of two oxygen atoms combined to make an oxygen molecule. If three oxygen atoms combine, an ozone molecule is formed. See Figure 6.

Ozone is also found high above the Earth in a layer called the stratosphere. That ozone is essential to life on Earth because it shields us from harmful ultraviolet B radiation from the sun. But when ozone forms near the ground, we have a very different situation.

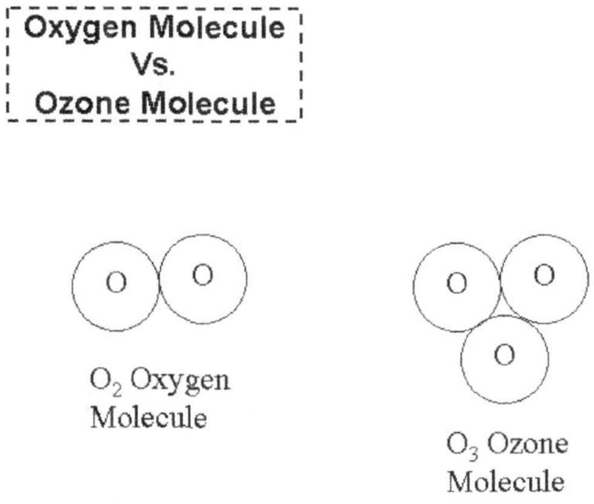

Figure 6. Oxygen and Ozone Molecules

Ground ozone forms when hydrocarbons react with sunlight and heat. See Figure 7. Smog is substantially ozone. This low altitude ozone is dangerous because it irritates the lungs and throat, which is a serious concern for asthma patients who already have inflamed airways.

There are two reasons for discussing ozone. First, you will actually find it produced by devices marketed to asthma victims! The marketers claim that their ozone is beneficial to asthma sufferers because it removes air impurities. Folks, ozone is still ozone. You should never use any device that produces ozone directly or indirectly. Ozone can cause permanent lung damage.

If the device is an ion generator or ozone generator, keep your money and your health. Many manufacturers will not explicitly state that ozone is produced. Some may use the words "active oxygen" or "plasma" instead of ozone. Be sure to investigate a device thoroughly before purchasing it. Both the Environmental Protection Agency (EPA) and the American Lung Association are strongly against the use of home ozone devices. Don't buy a device that will actually increase your lung damage!

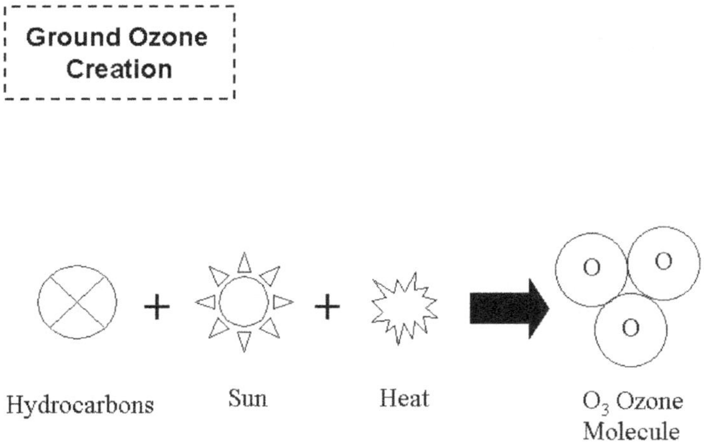

Figure 7. Ground Ozone Creation

The only safe air cleaners are those with a HEPA (High Efficiency Particulate Air) filter and no other electronic or ultraviolet processing. They produce no ozone. A HEPA filter can typically remove 99.97% of particles as small as 0.3 microns.

Now that we've covered this important side issue, let's return to ground ozone. It is a fact that ozone can induce asthma, so we need to find natural ways to combat this asthma trigger. Researchers found that ozone increases neutrophils and inflammatory cytokines in bronchoalveolar lavage fluid. Oxidative damage also occurs. The result is airway inflammation.[2, 10]

One study exposed participants to 0.12 ppm (parts per million) of ozone while exercising moderately. They also inhaled 0.10 ppm and 0.25 ppm of sulfur dioxide for 10 minutes.[2, 10]

The study found help from two of our support supplements. Vitamin E (400 IU) and vitamin C (500 mg) controlled the bronchial hyper-responsiveness in adult asthma patients. Those with more severe asthma were protected the most. Vitamin E was in the form of alpha tocopherol.[2, 10]

The researchers also made an interesting comment about the unexplained increase in asthma among persons under 18 years of age. They said that it would be interesting to examine the antioxidant status and effects of supplememtation on ozone-induced bronchial hyper-responsiveness in asthmatic children.[2, 10]

Could it be that children do not get enough antioxidants because of poor eating habits? If junk food has replaced fresh fruits and vegetables, they will lack the necessary ozone defenses such as vitamin E and C. Furthermore, how many children take good vitamin and mineral supplements? Could appropriate supplemenation help these children? I believe it would. It helped the adults in the study.

PESTICIDES AND ASTHMA

In the previous section we examined the role that ozone plays in asthma problems. You may be familiar with "ozone alerts" that are issued in many urban areas. Have you ever heard of a "pesticide alert"? Perhaps there should be one according to the following research studies.

Several different types of insecticides, such as organophosphates, carbamates, pyrethrins and synthetic pyrethroids, have been linked to asthma.[3, 4]

The 2003 Children's Health Study found that children were ten times more likely to develop early and persistent asthma if they were exposed to herbicides before the age of one as compared to controls.[5] There is also a financial burden associated with asthma. The estimated annual cost to treat asthmatic Americans less than 18 years old is $3.2 billion. A severe asthma patient could spend as much as $12,800 per year on treatments.[6]

So, what should you do to protect yourself and your family? One thing you can do is not put dangerous pesticides on your lawn and garden, especially if you have children. It may save your children a lot of suffering and save your pocket book, too. Only eat organic certified, pesticide-free fruits and vegetables.

The pesticide problem applies to both meat-eaters and to vegetarians, but vegetarians may be at greater risk. They also face another risk that most meat-eaters do not.

Vegetarians believe in their healthy diet. In many ways they are correct. But a vegetarian diet lacks sufficient vitamin B-12 unless dairy products and eggs are consumed. Vitamin B-12 is required to activate folate, another B vitamin. Both vitamin B-12 and folate are needed to convert dangerous homocysteine into methionine. What's the big deal? Homocysteine causes atherosclerosis, which is a hardening or thickening of the arteries. It results in plaque being built up inside arteries that could break off and cause a stroke or heart attack.[11]

What's a vegetarian to do? Supplement your diet with vitamin B-12. See the vitamin B-12 section earlier in this book for details on what form of B-12 to use and how much. Still take a MVM to insure high enough levels of all vitamins and by all means eat only organically grown, fresh fruits and vegetables.

THE ALLERGY FOOD CHAIN

We already chewed on the vegetarians, so now let's square off with the carnivorous T Rex types.

People who eat lots of red meat have their own set of problems. Meat that is heavy in saturated fats, hormones, antibiotics and pesticides constitutes a health disaster. Meat also contains high amounts of omega-6 fatty acids (linoleic acid) and it is here we begin the allergy trail.

The body converts omega-6 fatty acids into arachidonic acid. This acid is the building block for the inflammatory chemicals involved in allergy and asthma reactions.[12]

Excessive intake of omega 6 fatty acids starts a chain reaction of events. More omega-6 means more arachidonic acid is produced. More arachidonic acid produces more eicosanoids (prostaglandins and leukotrienes), which produce more Th2 immune cells, which produce more IgE.[12] Remember, IgE is a key substance (remember the mast cell) directly involved in allergic reactions. The result is an increased chance for an inflammatory response (Figure 8). That increases your risk for an allergic reaction or asthma attack.

Omega-3 fatty acids (alpha-linoleic acid) limit eicosanoid production. If leukotrienes and inflammatory prostaglandins are reduced, asthmatic reactions can be reduced.[7]

Omega-3 is found in fatty fish like salmon. You need to tip the balance in favor of omega-3 versus omega-6. You can do this by taking fish oil capsules and by eating certain fish (without ingested mercury). See the discussion on fish oil in an earlier chapter.

A study also showed that toddlers are twice as likely to develop asthma if they eat large amounts of margarine and foods fried in vegetable oil as compared to children who do not. Margarine and vegetable oils contain polyunsaturated fats, which increase omega-6 fatty acids.

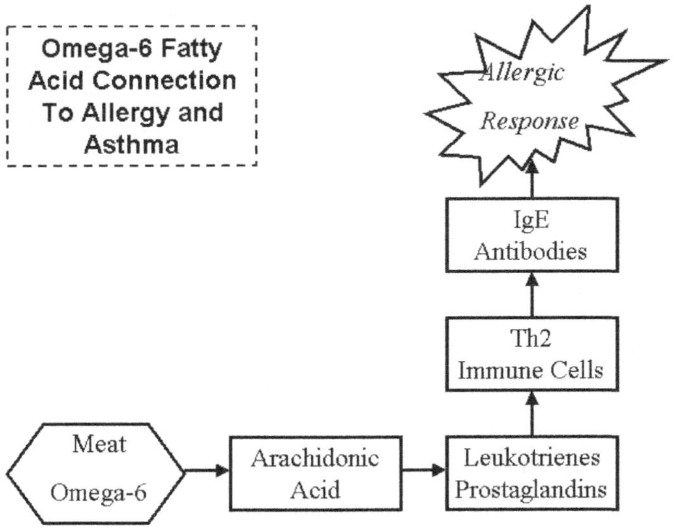

Figure 8. Meat and Allergy Connection

The authors concluded that polyunsaturated fat accounted for about 17% of the asthma cases in the study and another 16% were due to not breast-feeding.[8]

Omega-6 fatty acid content is not the only problem with meat. Frequently, it is loaded with antibiotics and pesticides. Pesticides were already discussed. How do antibiotics fit into the allergy picture? Antibiotics kill the body's natural flora or good bacteria, which live in the gut. This flora is absolutely essential to health.[13]

Have ever heard the term leaky gut syndrome? It refers to incompletely digested foods, bacteria and toxins that leak through the gut wall. They eventually find their way into the blood stream and cause an immune system response. The inflammatory response can result in allergies or asthma. Here is a partial list of leaky gut factors: [13]

- Tobacco
- Alcohol

- Antibiotics & other drugs
- Refined sugar
- Refined flour
- Food preservatives
- Caffeine
- Mercury (from fish and dental fillings)
- Aspirin
- Ibuprofen

Since we are talking about meat, let's zero in on antibiotics. Most cattle are treated with antibiotics. Ranchers want more of their cattle to survive diseases, so they give them plenty of antibiotics. The more cattle they have to sell, the more money they make. It's simple economics.

There are two problems with this, however. People who eat the beef also ingest the antibiotic remnants. Constant use of antibiotics causes germs to mutate into forms that are antibiotic resistant. When we really need an antibiotic to stop a bacterial (not viral) infection, it may not work. The germs may have mutated to defend themselves against that particular antibiotic.

Antibiotic-resistant bacteria have already have become a serious problem due to the over-prescription by many physicians. Many times a patient will get an antibiotic even though the problem is a viral infection. Antibiotics are worthless against a virus.

A second problem is the link with allergies and asthma. Researchers at the University of Michigan Medical School found that antibiotics may be responsible for killing good bacteria or flora, in the gut. Fungi then took over control of the gut. The fungi produce oxylipins, which are molecules that determine the kind of immune response and how severe it will be. The oxylipins resisted the production of regulatory T cells for ingested allergens. [9]

The respiratory T cells then became vulnerable to allergens such as mold spores and pollen. All of these actions combined produce an allergic response. In some cases they produce asthma.[9]

So does all this mean that we should not eat meat? No, but we should balance our consumption of meats, fruits and vegetables. Over consumption of any one food group at the expense of others is not wise. Substitute mercury-free fish in place of some of the red meat in your diet to reduce your omega-6 intake. Another good choice is poultry that is free of hormones and pesticides.

You can also buy different meat. Certified organic beef is free of pesticides, hormones and antibiotics. Feedlot cattle, on the other hand, are fed grain diets laced with antibiotics and hormones to get them to market much quicker. Grain is not the natural food for cattle. Grass is. Organic beef is leaner and much healthier.

The only catch is that you will have to pay more for certified organic beef, but you may pay less in medical bills. You weigh the cost-benefits. Regardless if you are a vegetarian or a meat and potatoes person, eating foods free of pesticides, hormones and antibiotics is absolutely necessary for a healthy life.

Natural supplements just give you a higher concentration of certain healthy ingredients found in organically certified foods. The higher concentrations are necessary to overcome existing medical conditions such as allergies and asthma. You would have to eat too much in order to get therapeutic doses from fruits and vegetables. Obesity is not a good option. The solution is to eat right as well as take the appropriate natural supplements to overcome those nasty medical conditions that plague you. If you are healthy, then just eating right may be all you need to do.

CHAPTER 7

THE FDA ON TRIAL

The *Food and Drug Administration* is supposed to protect the public and keep it healthy. This agency has a woeful track record. In addition to approving many dangerous drugs, the FDA has tried mightily to keep natural supplement information from the public. You don't believe it? It was proven in federal court! Not once, but twice.[1, 8]

Before the court decisions against the FDA, it was illegal to describe how any supplement could provide a health benefit. A bottle of Boswellia, for example, could not state that it supports joint health and mobility. The FDA required almost total proof before it would allow any health claims for either supplements or foods.[8]

This policy was absolutely detrimental to the health of the American public. Information that would help people conquer diseases and live healthier, longer lives was banished. Disobedience by a manufacturer resulted in an unannounced visit by the U.S. Marshals.

THE PEARSON I CASE

Two court cases were instrumental in restoring our First Amendment rights. The first came in 1999 with the case of Pearson vs. Shalala (Pearson I). The suit stated that the FDA refused to allow these four claims: [8]

1. "Consumption of antioxidant vitamins may reduce the risk of certain kinds of cancers."
2. "Consumption of fiber may reduce the risk of colorectal cancer."
3. "Consumption of omega-3 fatty acids may reduce the risk of coronary heart disease."
4. ".8 mg of folic acid in a dietary supplement is more effective in reducing the risk of neural tube defects than a lower amount in foods in common form."[2]

The judge ordered the FDA to allow the statement "Consumption of antioxidant vitamins may reduce the risk of certain kinds of cancers" with the disclaimer "These statement have not been evaluated by the Food and Drug Administration." Guess what happened? The arrogant FDA refused to comply with the order! [8]

THE PEARSON II CASE

Then, in 2002, the FDA lost a second court decision in a suit filed by Dr. Julian Whitaker and others (Pearson II). Judge Gladys Kessler of the United States District Court for the District of Columbia ruled that the FDA's actions violated the free speech clause of the Constitution. The FDA was convicted a second time for illegal censorship.[3, 8]

The court said, "The scientific consensus, even as acknowledged by the FDA, confirms that taking folic acid substantially reduces a woman's risk of giving birth to an infant with a neural tube defect. The public interest is well served by permitting information about the ability of folic acid to reduce the risk of neural tube defects to reach as wide a public audience as possible." [8]

The FDA had lost its illegal power to ban health claims of nutritional supplements unless it had actual evidence that the claims were false.

Just think of the harm that the FDA had inflicted on the American public for so many years. But that was not enough. The FDA deliberately disobeyed the court for two years after losing Pearson I and only relented after losing a second lawsuit.[8]

How many people would not have died of cancer or heart disease had the FDA allowed the first three claims in Pearson I? How many unborn children would not have been harmed if the FDA had permitted claim number four in Pearson I? How many died in the two years of non-compliance? Today, good doctors tell expectant mothers to take folic acid to prevent birth defects – but no thanks to the FDA.[8, 9]

After their second defeat, the FDA created the "Better Health Information for Consumers" policy to comply with the Pearson I and Pearson II edicts. It was really damage control, and it was not voluntary.[4, 5, 6, 8]

Someday supplement manufacturers might make claims about their nutriceuticals in much the same way that pharmaceutical companies do about their drugs.[7, 8] The legal fights continue, however.[1, 9]

CONCLUSION

Now let's review the facts:

FACT: Prescription drugs cause considerable harm each year (see chapter 1).

FACT: the FDA approves all drugs.

FACT: The FDA has repeatedly hindered the use of natural supplements to fight disease.

FACT: The FDA has ignored federal court decisions and continued illegal activities against natural supplements, which resulted in dire consequences for the public, including babies.

CONCLUSION: You decide if the FDA is the public's friend or foe. You decide who the FDA puts first – the American public or the pharmaceutical-medical complex.

The FDA assumes that only drugs can treat diseases. Natural treatments have been used for thousands of years. The drug industry has been around for less than a 100 years. How did mankind survive all that time without the drug companies and the FDA?

The roadblocks and harassment of the FDA regarding the benefits of natural alternatives should and must stop. Scientific evidence to support such benefits should not be ignored because no drug was involved. It should also not take hundreds of millions of dollars to prove a natural health claim.

The drug companies have an allegiance to their stockholders. The pharmaceutical industry has numerous registered lobbyists in Washington and spends hundreds of millions of dollars in political contributions. Neither Congress nor the FDA should succumb to the pressures of big-business lobbyists at the expense of the American public.

The FDA should have an allegiance to the American people, and not to the pharmaceutical-medical complex. Lip service is not enough. Immediate compliance with the U.S. Constitution and rulings by the federal courts are mandatory, but only the beginning of a complete attitude change that is necessary to truly protect the health of America.

Finally, I wish to reiterate my position from chapter one. I am all for the use of pharmaceuticals in emergency situations and when there are no alternatives available. They definitely can save lives. I am against their continuous use when safe, natural alternatives exist. This is especially true in the long-term management of a medical condition.

Each person is ultimately responsible for his or her own health. You need to be well informed in order to successfully meet your health challenges. I hope that you have found this book informative and practical. I wish you good health – the natural way!

APPENDIX A

Just as I strongly believe in the natural approach to healing whenever possible, I also believe that I should share with you the best news of all – how you can go to Heaven and KNOW that are going there for sure. This is God's Gospel, or Good News, as given in the *Bible (KJV)*. Please take a few moments to read it.

►God will not allow any sinners into Heaven. The dilemma is that everyone is a sinner.

"If we say that we have no sin, we deceive ourselves, and the truth is not in us." (1 John 1:8)

"All we like sheep have gone astray; we have turned every one to his own way; and the LORD hath laid on him the iniquity of us all." (Isaiah. 53:6)

►The Penalty of sin is death and eternal separation from God.

"For the wages of sin [is] death; but the gift of God [is] eternal life through Jesus Christ our Lord." (Romans 6:23)

►You can't earn your salvation or work your way into Heaven.

"For by grace are ye saved through faith; and that not of yourselves: [it is] the gift of God: Not of works, lest any man should boast." (Ephesians 2:8,9)

"Therefore we conclude that a man is justified by faith without the deeds of the law." (Romans 3:28)

"Not by works of righteousness which we have done, but according to his mercy he saved us, by the washing of regeneration, and renewing of the Holy Ghost; Which he shed on us abundantly through Jesus Christ our Saviour; That being justified by his grace, we should be made heirs according to the hope of eternal life." (Titus 3:5-7)

►Jesus Christ paid for ALL our sins – past, present and future – when He died on the cross; therefore, we can be righteous (sinless) in the sight of God.

"For he hath made him [to be] sin for us, who knew no sin; that we might be made the righteousness of God in him." (2Corinthians 5:21)

"... and the LORD hath laid on him the iniquity of us all." (Isaiah. 53:6)

►God will only see you as sinless if you believe that Jesus Christ died to pay for all your sins, was buried and rose again on the third day. If you accept His payment for your sins, He gives you the FREE GIFT OF ETERNAL LIFE IN HEAVEN!

"For God so loved the world, that he gave his only begotten Son, that whosoever believeth in him should not perish, but have everlasting life." (John 3:16)

"And brought them out, and said, Sirs, what must I do to be saved? And they said, Believe on the Lord Jesus Christ, and thou shalt be saved, and thy house." (Acts 16:30-31)

►You can KNOW that you are going to Heaven.

"These things have I written unto you that believe on the name of the Son of God; that ye may <u>know</u> that ye have eternal life, and that ye may believe on the name of the Son of God." (1 John 5:13)

"Verily, verily, I say unto you, He that believeth on me <u>hath</u> everlasting life." (John 6:47)

►You can NEVER lose your salvation. You have eternal security. The Bible says so.

"To an inheritance incorruptible, and undefiled, and that <u>fadeth not away</u>, reserved in heaven for you, Who are kept by the power of God through faith unto salvation ready to be revealed in the last time." (1 Peter 1:4-5)

"And I give unto them eternal life; and they shall <u>never</u> perish, neither shall any [man] pluck them out of my hand." (John 10:28)

"And this is the Father's will which hath sent me, that of all which he hath given me I should lose <u>nothing</u>, but should raise it up again at the last day." (John 6:39)

APPENDIX B

This appendix gives helpful suggestions on when to take the various supplements. Many depend on one or more additional supplements for absorption or effectiveness. Some supplements should not be taken at the same time because they interfere with each other.

The "two meal list" assumes that most people would be at work during lunch and would not take supplements then. I have also assumed that the MVM (multi-vitamin-mineral) requires two capsules per day for a normal daily dose. If yours requires three or more capsules per day, make the appropriate adjustment to spread them out over the day.

If you are able to take supplements with all three meals, then use the "three meal list".

All doses are for an adult. **For children, consult your doctor.** The general way to calculate child doses is by weight ratios. The adult dose is usually assumed to be for a 150 lb. person. A 100 lb. child (12 or older) would get ⅔ of an adult dose (100 lb/150 lb = ⅔).

A deciding factor for children supplementation is whether or not they can swallow pills. Some supplements, like Yamoa, come in either capsule or powder form. Train your child early to swallow pills. Start with a tiny one and work your way up to larger ones. Instruct them exactly how to do it. Don't assume that they know how.

ALWAYS start with the MINIMUM dose for any herbal supplement just in case you are allergic to the plant! After three days, increase your dose gradually to be safe.

Two Meal List

BREAKFAST

MVM dose # 1

Vitamin B-12 (methylcobalamin lozenge) 1000 mcg

Magnesium 400 – 500 mg

Vitamin C with Bioflavonoids 1000 – 2000 mg

Quercetin 400 mg

NAC 600 mg

Boswellia 300 mg

Pycnogenol® 100 mg

Rosmarinic Acid 100 mg

Luteolin 4 mg

Yamoa 500 mg

CoQ10 60 – 100 mg

SUPPER

MVM dose # 2

Calcium 500 – 750 mg

Vitamin C with Bioflavonoids 500 – 2000 mg

Quercetin 200 – 400 mg

Vitamin E 400 – 800 IU (count your MVM amount, too)

Fish Oil 1500 – 4000 mg

Boswellia 300 mg

Lycopene 15 – 30 mg

Yamoa 500 mg

CoQ10 60 – 100 mg

Three Meal List

BREAKFAST

MVM dose # 1, one of two

Vitamin B-12 (methylcobalamin lozenge) 1000 mcg

Magnesium 200 – 250 mg

Vitamin C with Bioflavonoids 1000 – 2000 mg

Quercetin 200 – 400 mg

NAC 600 mg

Boswellia dose 300 mg

Rosmarinic Acid 100 mg

Luteolin 4 mg

Yamoa 500 mg

CoQ10 60 – 100 mg

LUNCH

Boswellia 300 mg

CoQ10 60 – 100 mg

Pycnogenol® 100 mg

Lycopene 15 –30 mg

Vitamin C with Bioflavonoids 500 – 1000 mg

Quercetin 200 – 400 mg

Magnesium 200 – 250 mg

Calcium 200 – 250 mg

SUPPER

MVM dose # 2, two of two

Calcium 250 – 500 mg

Vitamin C with Bioflavonoids 500 – 1000 mg

Quercetin 200 – 400 mg

NAC 600 mg (optional)

Vitamin E 400 – 800 IU (count your MVM amount, too)

Fish Oil 1500 – 4000 mg

Boswellia 300 mg

Yamoa 500 mg

CoQ10 60 – 100 mg

Rosmarinic Acid 100 mg (optional)

Luteolin 4 mg (optional)

APPENDIX C

My Personal Supplement Plan

BREAKFAST

Supplement	**Dose**	**Date Started**

LUNCH

Supplement	Dose	Date Started

SUPPER

Supplement	**Dose**	**Date Started**

APPENDIX D

Progress Diary

<u>Week # 1</u>

Acute Attack: ______________________________

Symptoms: ________________________________

____

____

____

____

____

____

____

____

____

____

____

____

Week # 2

Acute Attack: ______________________________

Symptoms: ______________________________

____

____

____

____

____

____

____

____

____

____

____

____

<u>Week # 3</u>

Acute Attack: ____________________________________

Symptoms: ______________________________________

____

____

____

____

____

____

____

____

____

____

____

____

Week # 4

Acute Attack: ______________________________________

Symptoms: ____

____

____

____

____

____

____

____

____

____

____

____

____

Week # 5

Acute Attack: ________________________________

Symptoms: __________________________________

____

____

____

____

____

____

____

____

____

____

____

____

Week # 6

Acute Attack: ______________________________________

Symptoms: ____

____

____

____

____

____

____

____

____

____

____

____

____

Week # 7

Acute Attack: ________________________________

Symptoms: ________________________________

____

____

____

____

____

____

____

____

____

____

____

____

Week # 8

Acute Attack: ____________________________________

Symptoms: ______________________________________

____

____

____

____

____

____

____

____

____

____

____

____

Week # 9

Acute Attack: ________________________________

Symptoms: __________________________________

____

____

____

____

____

____

____

____

____

____

____

____

Week # 10

Acute Attack: ______________________________________

Symptoms: ____

____

____

____

____

____

____

____

____

____

____

____

____

Week # 11

Acute Attack: ___________________________________

Symptoms: _____________________________________

____

____

____

____

____

____

____

____

____

____

____

____

Week # 12

Acute Attack: ______________________________________

Symptoms: ____

____

____

____

____

____

____

____

____

____

____

____

____

Week # 13

Acute Attack: ________________________________

Symptoms: __________________________________

____

____

____

____

____

____

____

____

____

____

____

____

Week # 14

Acute Attack: ____

Symptoms: ____

____

____

____

____

____

____

____

____

____

____

____

____

Week # 15

Acute Attack: ___________________________________

Symptoms: _____________________________________

____

____

____

____

____

____

____

____

____

____

____

____

Week # 16

Acute Attack: ________________________________

Symptoms: __________________________________

____

____

____

____

____

____

____

____

____

____

____

____

NOTES

CHAPTER 1

WHY GO NATURAL?

1. Garbe E, et al. Association of inhaled corticosteroid use with cataract extraction in elderly patients. *JAMA*, 1998;vol. 280, no. 6.

2. McKeever TM, Lewis SA, Smit HA, Burney P, Britton JR, Cassano PA. The association of acetaminophen, aspirin, and ibuprofen with respiratory disease and lung function. *Am J Resp Crit Care Med*. 2005 May 1;171(9):966-71.

3. Lazarou J, et al. Incidence of adverse drug reactions in hospitalized patients. *JAMA*. 1998;279(15):1200-5.

4. Miller III ER, et al. Meta-Analysis: High-Dosage Vitamin E Supplementation May Increase All-Cause Mortality. *Annals of Internal Medicine. 2005* Jan 4;Volume 142:Issue 1.

CHAPTER 2

MEET THE ENEMY

1. *Life Extension Disease Prevention and Treatment Expanded Fourth Edition*. 2003;pp. 39-40.

2. Costa JJ, Welker PF, Galli SJ. The cells of the allergic response: mast cells, basophils, and eosinophils. *JAMA.* 1997 Dec 10;278(22):1815-22.

3. Wong BR, Grossbard EB, Payan DG, Masuda ES. Targeting Syk as a treatment for allergic and autoimmune disorders. *Expert Opin Investing Drugs.* 2004 Jul;13(7):743-62.

4. Bavbeck S, Demiral YS, Erekul S, Kalayctoglu O, Beder S, Misirligil Z, Gurbuz L. The mechanism of bronchial hyperactivity in allergic rhinitis patients. *Allergol Immunopathol [Madr].* 1996 Mar-Apr;24(2):45-53.

5. Ciprandi G, Cirill I, Vizzaccaro A, Milanese M, Tosca MA. Airway function and nasal inflammation in seasonal allergic rhinitis and asthma. *Clin Exp Allergy.* 2004 Jun;34(6):891-6.

6. Leung SY, Eynott P, Noble A, Nath P, Chung KF. Resolution of allergic airways inflammation but persistence of airway smooth muscle proliferation after repeated allergen exposures. *Clin Exp Allergy.* 2004 Feb;34(2):213-20.

7. Storms WW. Exercise-induced asthma: diagnosis and treatment for the recreational or elite athlete. *Med Sci Sports Exerc.* 1999;31(suppl 1):S33-S38.

8. Colman J. Rosmarinic Acid Provides Natural Allergy Relief. *LifeExtension Collector's Edition 2005*. p. 144.

9. Ibid., p. 147.

CHAPTER 3

THE NATURAL ARSENAL PART I

1. Ames B, et al. High-dose vitamin therapy stimulates variant enzymes with decreased coenzyme binding affinity (increased Km): relevance to genetic disease and polymorphisms. *Am J Clin Nutr.* 2002;75:616-58.

2. Neuman I, Nahum H, Ben-Amotz A. Prevention of exercise-induced asthma by a natural isomer mixture of beta-carotene. *Ann Allerg Asthma Immunol.* 1999;82:549–53.

3. Collipp PJ, Goldzier S III, Weiss N, et al. Pyridoxine treatment of childhood bronchial asthma. *Ann Allergy.* 1975;35:93–7.

4. Reynolds RD, Natta CL. Depressed plasma pyridoxal phosphate concentrations in adult asthmatics. *Am J Clin Nutr.* 1985;41:684–8.

5. Sur S, Camara M, Buchmeier A, et al. Double-blind trial of pyridoxine (vitamin B-6) in the treatment of steroid-dependent asthma. *Ann Allergy.* 1993;70:141–52.

6. Anibarro B, Caballero T, Garcia-Ara C, et al. Asthma with sulfite intolerance in children: A blocking study with cyanocobalamin. *J Allergy Clin Immunol.* 1992;90:103–9.

7. Forastiere F, Pistelli R, Sestini P, et al. Consumption of fresh fruit rich in vitamin C and wheezing symptoms in children. SIDRIA Collaborative Group, Italy (Italian Studies on Respiratory Disorders in Children and the Environment). *Thorax.* 2000;55:283–8.

8. Zuskin E, Valic F, Bouhuys A. Byssinosis and airway responses due to exposure to textile dust. *Lung.* 1976;154:17–24.

9. Bucca C, Rolla G, Oliva A, Farina J-C. Effect of vitamin C on histamine bronchial responsiveness of patients with allergic rhinitis. *Ann Allergy.* 1990;65:311–4.

10. Anah CO, Jarike LN, Baig HA. High dose ascorbic acid in Nigerian asthmatics. *Trop Geogr Med.* 1980;32:132–7.

11. Centanni S et al. The potential role of tocopherol in asthma and allergies: modification of the leukotriene pathway. *BioDrugs.* 2001;15(2):81-86.

12. Fogarty, A et al. Dietary vitamin E, IgE concentrations, and atopy. *Lancet.* 2000;356:1573-4.

13. Haury VG. Blood serum magnesium in bronchial asthma and its treatment by the administration of magnesium sulfate. *J Lab Clin Med.* 1940;26:340–4.

14. Skobeloff EM, Spivey WH, McNamara RM, Greenspon L. Intravenous magnesium sulfate for the treatment of acute asthma in the emergency department. *JAMA.* 1989;262:1210–3.

15. Hill J, Micklewright A, Lewis S, Britton J. Investigation of the effect of short-term change in dietary magnesium intake in asthma. *Eur Respir J.* 1997;10:2225–9.

16. Hill J, et al. Investigation of the effect of short-term change in dietary magnesium intake in asthma. *Eur Respir J.* 1997;10:2225-9.

17. Bede O, et al. Urinary magnesium excretion in asthmatic children receiving magnesium supplementation: randomized, placebo-controlled, double-blind study. *Magnes Res.* 2003;16:262-70.

18. Stone J, Hinks LJ, Beasley R, et al. Reduced selenium status of patients with asthma. *Clin Sci.* 1989;77:495–500.

19. Flatt A, Pearce N, Thomson CD, et al. Reduced selenium in asthmatic subjects in New Zealand. *Thorax.* 1990;45:95–9.

20. Kadrabova J, Mad'aric A, Kovacikova Z, et al. Selenium status is decreased in patients with intrinsic asthma. *Biol Trace Elem Res.* 1996;52:241–8.

21. Misso NL, Powers KA, Gillon RL, et al. Reduced platelet glutathione peroxidase activity and serum selenium concentration in atopic asthmatic patients. *Clin Exp Allergy.* 1996;26:838–47.

22. *Life Extension Disease Prevention and Treatment Expanded Fourth Edition*. 2003;p.140.

23. Ibid., p. 41.

24. Hasselmark L, Malmgren R, Zetterstrom O, Unge G. Selenium supplementation in intrinsic asthma. *Allergy* 1993;48:30–6.

CHAPTER 4

THE NATURAL ARSENAL PART II

1. Uz T, et al. Aging-associated up-regulation of neuronal 5-lipoxygenase expression: putative role in neuronal vulnerability. *FASEB.* 1998;12:439-49.

2. Gupta I, et al. Effects of Boswellia serrata gum resin in patients with bronchial asthma: results of a double-blind, placebo-controlled, 6 week clinical study. *Eur J Med Res.* 1998;3:511-14.

3. Fogarty A, Britton J. The role of diet in the aetiology of asthma. *Clin Exp Allergy.* 2000;30:615–27.

4. Arm JP, Horton CE, Eiser NM, et al. The effects of dietary supplementation with fish oil on asthmatic responses to antigen. *J Allergy Clin Immunol.* 1988;81:183 [abstract #57].

5. Broughton KS, Johnson CS, Pace BK, et al. Reduced asthma symptoms with n-3 fatty acid ingestion are related to 5-series leukotriene production. *Am J Clin Nutr.* 1997;65:1011–7.

6. Hodge L, Salome CM, Peat JK, et al. Consumption of oily fish and childhood asthma risk. *Med J Austral.* 1996;164:137–40.

7. Nagakura T, Matsuda S, Shichijyo K, et al. Dietary supplementation with fish oil rich in omega-3 polyunsaturated fatty acids in children with bronchial asthma. *Eur Respir. J* 2000;16:861–5.

8. Neuman I, Nahum H, Ben-Amotz A. Reduction of exercise-induced asthma oxidative stress by lycopene, a natural antioxidant. *Allergy.* 2000;55:1184–9.

9. Bengtsson A, et al. Thiols decrease cytokine levels and down-regulate the expression of CD30 on human allergen-specific T helper (Th) 0 and Th2 cells. *Clin Exp Immunol.* 2001 Mar;123(3):350-60.

10. Rohdewald P. A review of the French maritime pine bark extract (Pycnogenol), a herbal medication with a diverse clinical pharmacology. *Internat J of Clin Pharmy and Therap.* 2002;40(4):158-168.

11. Quercetin (Monograph). *Alt Med. Rev* 3 1998:140-143.

12. Leighton T, University California Berkeley Quercetin Project (preliminary report). 1988.

13. Pearce F, et al. Mucosal mast cells III. Effect of quercetin and other flavonoids on antigen-induced histamine secretion from rat intestinal mast cells. *J Allergy Clin Immunol.* 73 1984:819-23.

14. Middleton E, et al. Quercetin: an inhibitor of antigen-induced human basophil histamine release. *J Immunol.* 127 1981:546-50.

15. Foreman J. Mast cells and actions of flavonoids. *J Allergy Clin Immunol.* 73 1984:769-73.

16. Middleton E, et al. The effects of plant flavonoids on mammalian cells: implications for inflammation, heart disease and cancer. *Pharmacol Rev.* 52 2000:673-751.

17. Life Extension Disease Prevention and Treatment Expanded Fourth Edition. 2003; pp. 41-42.

18. Ibid., p. 141.

19. Klegeris A, et al. Cyclooxygenase and 5 lipooxygenase inhibitors protect against mononuclear

phagocyte neurotoxicity. *Neurobiol of Aging* 2002 (23) 787-794.

CHAPTER 5

SUPER, NATURAL WEAPONS

1. Takano H, Osakabe N, Sanbongi C, et al. Extract of Perilla frutescens enriched for rosmarinic acid inhibits seasonal allergic rhinoconjunctivitis in humans. *Exp Bio Med.* 2004 Mar;229(3):247-54.

2. Hur YG, Yun Y, Won J. Rosmarinic acid induces p561ck-dependent apoptosis in jurkat and peripheral T cells via mitochondrial pathway independent from fas/fas ligand intertaction. *J Immunol.* 2004 Jan 1;172(1):79-87.

3. Yun SY, Hur YG, Kang MA, Lee J, Ahn C, Won J. Synergistic immunosuppressive effects of rosmarinic acid and rapamycin in vitro and in vivo. *Transplantation.* 2003 May 27;75(10):1758-60.

4. Sanbongi C, Takano H, Osakabe N. Rosmarinic acid inhibits lung injury induced by diesel exhaust particles. *Free Radic Biol Med.* 2003 Apr;15:34(8):1060-9.

5. Won J, Hur YG, Hur EM, et al. Rosmarinic acid inhibits TCR-induced T cell activation and proliferation in an Lck-dependent manner. *Eur J Immunal.* 2003 Apr;33(4):870-9.

6. Hu G, Walls RS, Bass D, et al. The Chinese herbal formulation Biminne in management of perennial allergic rhinitis: a randomized, double-blinded, placebo-controlled, 12 week clinical trial. *Ann Allergy Asthma Immunol.* 2002 May;88(5):478-87.

7. Borchers At, Sakai S, Henderson GL, et al. Shosaiko-to and other Kampo [Japanese herbal] medicines: a review of their immunomodulatory activities. *J Ethnopharmacol.* 2000 Nov;73(1-2):1-13.

8. Hirano T, Higa S, Arimitsu J, et al. Flavonoids such luteolin, fiseten, apigenin are inhibitors of interleukin-4 and interleukin-13 production by activated human basophils. *Int Arch Allergy Immunol.* 2004 Jun;134(2):135-40.

9. Park KY, Lee SH, Min BK, et al. Inhibitory effect of luteolin 4'-O-glucoside from Kummerowia striata and other flavonoids on interleukin-5 bioactivity. *Planta Med.* 1999 Jun;65(5):457-9.

10. Kimata M, et al. Effects of luteolin and other flavonoids on IgE-meditated allergic reactions. *Planta Med.* 2000;66:25-29.

11. Ueda H et al. Luteolin as an anti-inflammatory and anti-allergy constituent of *Perilla frutescens*. *Bio Pharm Bull.* 2002;25:1197-1202.

12. Colman J. Rosmarinic Acid Provides Natural Allergy Relief. *LifeExtension Collector's Edition 2005*. p. 144.

13. Ibid., p. 145.

14. Ibid., p. 146.

15. All Yamoa information used with permission from Yamoa.com.

CHAPTER 6

GARBAGE IN, DISEASE OUT

1. Andersen-Parrado P. With every breath we take, asthma is on the rise – but there is hope. *Better Nutrition.* 1997 Feb.

2. Trenga C, et al. Dietary Antioxidants and Ozone-Induced Bronchial Hyperresponsiveness in Adults with Asthma. *Archives of Environmental Health.* 2001 May.

3. Reigart JR, Roberts JR. Recognition and Management of Pesticide Poisonings, Fifth Edition. *U.S. EPA.* 1999 March;735-R-98-003.

4. Underner M, Cazenave F, Patte F. 1987. Occupational asthma in the rural environment. *Rev Pneumonol Clin*. 43:26-35.

5. Salam, MT, Y-F Li, B Langholz and FD Gilliland. Early Life Environmental Risk Factors for Asthma: Findings from the Children's Health Study. *Env Health Persp*. 2003;112:760-65.

6. Cisternas, et al. A Comprehensive Study of the Direct and Indirect Costs of Adult Asthma. *J Allergy Clin Immun*. 2003;111:1212-1218.

7. Kankaanpaa P, Sutas Y, Salminen S, Lichtenstein A & Isolauri E. Dietary fatty acids and allergy. *Ann Med*. 1999;31:282–287.

8. M M Haby, J K Peat, G B Marks, A J Woolcock, S R Leeder. Asthma in preschool children: prevalence and risk factors. *Thorax*. 2001 August;56:589-595.

9. Noverr MC, Nicole R. Falkowski NC, McDonald RA, McKenzie AN, Huffnagle GB. Development of Allergic Airway Disease in Mice following Antibiotic Therapy and Fungal Microbiota Increase: Role of Host Genetics, Antigen, and Interleukin-13. *Infection and Immunity*. 2005 January; Vol. 73, No. 1:30-38.

10. *Life Extension Disease Prevention and Treatment Expanded Fourth Edition*. 2003;pp.142-143.

11. *Ibid.,* p.146.

12. Ibid., p.141.

13. Ibid., p. 43.

CHAPTER 7

THE FDA ON TRIAL

1. See web site www.emord.com/legal/.

2. See www.emord.com/legal/fdadecision.htm for Pearson I.

3. See www.emord.com/docs/Memo%20Opinion%202-2-011.pdf for Pearson II.

4. U.S. Food and Drug Administration. Dietary Supplement Enforcement Report. 2002 Dec. 18:1.

5. U.S. Food and Drug Administration. FDA News, FDA Announces Initiative to Provide Better Health Information for Consumers. 2002 Dec. 18:1.

6. See www.fda.gov for Consumer Health Information for Better Nutrition.

7. U.S. Food and Drug Administration. Guidance for Industry, Qualified Health Claims in the Labeling of Conventional Foods and Dietary Supplements. 2002 Dec. 18:1.

8. A New Day at FDA? *LifeExtension 2003 April.* pp. 32-33.

9. Ibid., p. 35.

INDEX

Made in the USA
Las Vegas, NV
14 March 2026

43624239R00059